My Life

–

My Food Journey
to a
Healthier Self

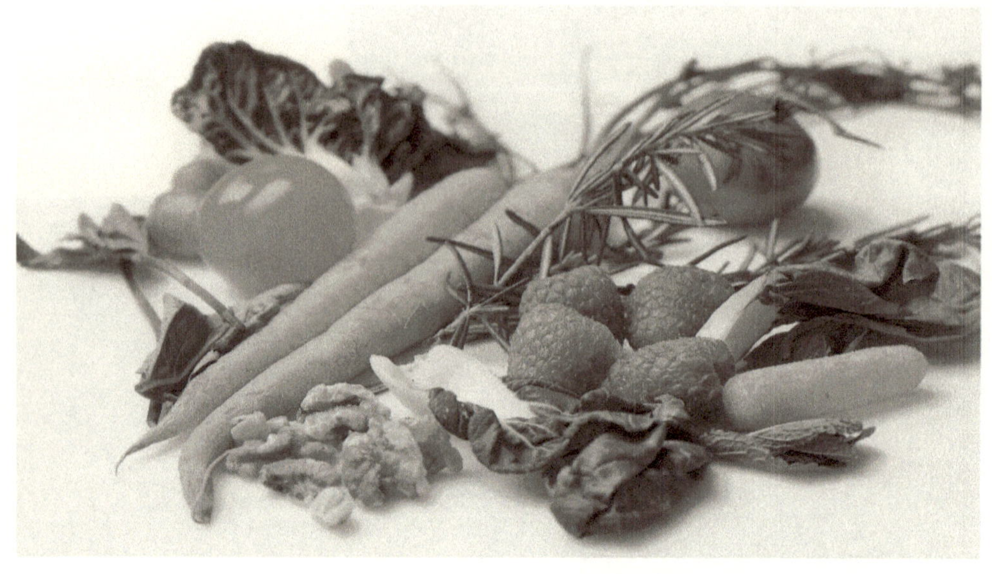

ISBN: 9781729314081
Imprint: Independently published

FIRST!

Thank you for purchasing *My Life – My Food Journal*.

You have taken the first step toward success. Now, let's get you moving forward by you deciding your success. I have a few questions for you.

What do you expect to achieve?

Are your plans realistic?

Do you plan to include exercise?

What impact will your food list have on your food budget?

How will you reward yourself when you reach your goal?

My Changing Body

First Month Challenge

Measurements	Week 1	Week 2	Week 3	Week 4
Neck				
Right Upper				
Left Upper Arm				
Right Wrist				
Left Wrist				
Chest				
Bust				
Midriff				
Natural Waist				
Abdomen				
Hips				
Buttocks				
Upper Thigh				
Middle Thigh				
Lower Thigh				
Above Knee				
Calf				
Ankle				
Starting				
Goal Weight				

As you progress through your journey, you will have ups and downs.

DO NOT get discouraged.

Change up your food selections, add a different type of exercise, and most of all –

Drink YOUR WATER!

Five Smart Trackable Ways to Weight Loss

Losing weight for many folks is such a struggle. Some can lose 5 pounds at the snap of your finger. However, some need to lose many more pounds: 30, 50, or as much as 100 or more pounds. This type of weight loss journey is not short and easy; it has many challenges, plateaus, and setbacks.

How can you accomplish this goal? Start with sensible goals and a plan. You will need dedication. Evan reaching a small goal is a win. Let's see what dedication breaks down into:

You are "HUMAN", I know, a real shocker!

We have many fallacies and that is just how we are made. Willpower can be short on supply when you are looking at your favorite Double Chocolate Chip Brownie. You will stumble in your weight loss journey, and that is the truth. However, the thing to do is stay focused on your overall goal.

Reasonable Goals Equals Success

Okay, you have a goal of 50 pounds or more to lose. That is awesome! Now, let's work out your PLAN. You can reach that goal by breaking it down to manageable steps.

Start by setting a goal of losing one to two pounds a week. Then take a very hard and honest look at your Meal Plan and Exercise Plan. Your Meal and Exercise plans work together.

How is that? First, you want to be able to keep the weight off. Starving one week and then binging the next is not healthy. And it will create a stumbling block. Losing one pound instead of two pounds is still a victory. It is one less pound your body must carry. It is a win.

Get a Friend to Help You

Deciding to start your Weight loss journey should never be done alone. One of the best motivators is competition and a workout partner makes the journey enjoyable. An app on your Smart Phone allows you to compete against yourself. A physical trainer can work with you and set goals for you to achieve. Of course, a nutritionist helps you to eat filling meals while still supporting your body nutritional requirements.

Overcome the Plateaus

As your weight changes, you will hit Plateaus. Do not give up. Change up what you are doing. Talk to your nutritionist to make sure you are eating healthy. Your trainer to change up your exercise routine. And of course, your doctor to get an overall check-up.

You may need to eat differently for a few days or weeks. Your exercise routine may need to change focus. And, you may have developed a health issue that was hidden before because of lack of activity.

Small Changes Equal Largest Successes

Have you heard the phrase, "It's all in the details"? Details are small, most of the time un-noticeable. In weight loss, small changes are capable of huge successes. For example, stairs instead of the elevator twice a week, flavored water instead of sweet tea or soda and fresh fruit for dessert instead of Double Chocolate Chip Brownie. I am not saying you cannot have a small piece of Double Chocolate Chip Brownie, once a week. Your goal is to create a Good Habit of selecting quality nutritious foods over bad. You want all this work to become a lifelong habit and get off the Weight Loss/Gain Train. Create a Good Habit that is enjoyable and healthy. Remember, long-term changes (6-12 weeks) create a lasting difference.

Boost Your Health - Fruits & Vegetables

Including fruits and vegetables in your daily diet will allow you to benefit from all the cell building value. You can enjoy these all year round. Some fruits are available only in the summer. However, you can still get some frozen/canned produce with no added sugar to enjoy. Let us begin with vegetables

Zucchini: Green or Yellow

This vegetable is about 95% water, Zero Fat, Zero Cholesterol, and very low in calories (about 20). Also, it helps control blood pressure, includes antioxidants and other nutrients like Vitamin C, Potassium, and Folate. You can easily add one cup of shredded Zucchini into your meals.

Sweet corn

This vegetable is naturally sweet, do not get it confused with Field Corn. Field Corn is mostly GMO's. And sweet corn has very important health benefits:

It helps your Vision with two phytochemicals: Zeaxanthin and lutein. During the cooking process, activity increases in antioxidants. It contains Ferulic Acid that helps fight cancer. The insoluble fiber helps keep you full longer and promotes weight loss. This vegetable is loaded with B Vitamins, iron, protein, and potassium. A medium sweet corn ear is only about 100 calories; this is without the butter. It is considered a "clean" food according to 2018 Environmental Working Group.

Tomatoes

Most consider tomatoes as a vegetable; however, it is a fruit. This high-powered vegetable can help reduce heart disease and cancer. They are loaded with Vitamin C, Vitamin K, and Potassium. A medium tomato only has about 18 calories, about 95% water, and contain about 5% fiber. They also include Beta-Carotene, Naringenin, Lycopene, and Chlorogenic Acid.

These red, yellow, orange vegetable have fighting abilities: Heart Health, Cancer Prevention, and Skin Health. Local tomatoes are better for you and are tasty. If you have access to a local farmer, you will have a better chance of finding vine ripe tomatoes. There is a huge difference in taste and quality.

String Beans

This vegetable is tasty and full of Potassium, Folate, Fiber, Iron, Zinc, and Protein. Also, string beans have Vitamin C, an infection fighter and immune booster. Even more important are the cancer fighting benefits and heart health antioxidants.

Sweet Potatoes

These tubers come in orange, deep purple, yellow, cream and almost white flesh, are naturally sweet and full of antioxidant nutrients. You can add a little "fat" to obtain the full beta-carotene benefits sweet potatoes are known for. The great benefits you will get when you add these tubers to your meal plan: Anti-inflammatory, Improves Blood Sugar control (even in type 2 diabetes), and Resin Glycosides.

Watermelons

The smell of watermelon brings smiles to everyone! With its Vitamin B6 to boost your mind, Lycopene, an antioxidant that fights attacks on your heart, cancer and eyes, you must take time to enjoy some of this wonderful fruit. It has Citrulline that increased blood flow, Vitamin C, Vitamin A, and is almost no fat.

Since this fruit is around 92% water, a hydrating food, it will reduce your hunger. Many times, we think we are hungry for food, when our body is starving for water.

As wonderful as this fruit is, it does come with two cautions. 1. Diabetics will have to watch how much they consume; especially, if on dialysis. 2. A natural diuretic when eaten on an empty stomach.

Stone Fruits: Apricots, Cherries, Nectarines, Peaches, and Plums

 Boost Immunity - These stone fruits are loaded with Vitamin C which helps to build a H3 immune system.

Healthy Skin Builder - Collagen, your body's most abundant protein, helps connective tissue structure.

Your Eye Health - Peaches, Nectarines, and Apricots each have an orange color which comes from the carotenoid content.

Heart Healthy - The fiber of these stone fruits may contribute to lower cholesterol levels and the antioxidants may protect your arteries and assist in achieving better blood pressure.

 GI Health - The stone fruit fiber helps to promote good digestive health. This fiber helps promote bowel movements, helps prevent digestive system cancers, and reduces hemorrhoid issues.

Increase Your Fat Burning Power - These stone fruits help you fight against diabetes, inflammatory issues, obesity, and what is called Metabolic Syndrome.

Cell Protection - Because of their phytochemical content, they protect your cells from damage. This can reduce your risk of developing specific types of cancers.

Cherry juice helps to reduce muscle pain with anti-inflammatory attributes. Cherries - high in Melatonin, helps to control your body's cycles for sleep and wake.

Peaches - Help reduce anxiety and promote relaxation, helping you sleep better.

Plums - The Vitamin K choice, this nutrient helps maintain healthy bones and teeth. Joins the fight against osteoporosis and osteoarthritis.

 These stone fruits are versatile: You can purchase them: fresh, frozen, canned, juice/nectar, or dried. Have a healthy snack ready when your real hunger pains attack.

Pineapples

High in bromelain - a proteolytic enzyme, pineapples help with the digestion process. They're also an excellent source of antioxidants, which means they ward off free radicals and protect the body from their harmful effects, while reducing the risk of serious inflammatory diseases.

Cherries

These round, succulent fruits color is a clear indication of how powerful its antioxidants are and how much protection they offer against heart disease, mainly due to their high levels of pectin which helps balance blood cholesterol levels. Cherries are also great health-boosters since they contain melatonin, which is known as **THE** "sleep hormone."

Melatonin is secreted naturally by the body during the night, but foods rich in melatonin can help induce a restful sleep. It's also a wide-spectrum, potent antioxidant. Moreover, melatonin helps with the conversion process of turning fat cells, which collect under our skin and around our organs, into brown fat cells, which work at burning calories instead of storing them.

Mangoes

Sweet and savory, mangoes pack a great amount of fiber, iron, magnesium, and antioxidants. They also help with the digestion process as well as curb your hunger by filling you up for longer.

Figs

These summer snacks are packed with potassium and fiber. They're also low in calories and fat.

Grapes

Like watermelon, grapes have a high-water content, which makes you feel full longer. They also help protect against disease, such as Type 2 diabetes; packed with antioxidants and inflammatory properties, phytochemicals and vitamin C.

Empowering You in Healthy Eating

Each day we accept things around us as reasonable and do nothing to change those things which do us the most harm. Although, it is in our face, we are totally blind. That is the way it has always been, so we see "no need" to make a change. Bad habits are so easy to create; they make us feel good. Eating a chocolate bar and drinking soda is so much easier than taking the time to fix a healthy meal.

Then, something happens in our lives that makes us step back and take a hard look at our life and our future. Stark reality sets in; we are sometimes shocked we have allowed ourselves to become embroiled in such a mess. Meanwhile, questioning our oversight. We want to put the blame on our current situation instead of accepting the responsibility for our own actions.

The environment we live in has the power to dictate our future if we become complacent and lazy. For example: We were raised getting doughnuts for breakfast each morning. As adults, we would think that behavior is normal. Our friends always wanted to have sleepovers because of the doughnuts for breakfast. Even though, we grow up and "see" other choices, the doughnuts are our excuse to continue with the action.

What if we never ate breakfast growing up? Then, we got married and our spouse was asking for breakfast?

Now what? How do we change?

It is easy! One breakfast at a time, period!

Food is our Achilles heel. To live we must consume it.

Sweets, fast foods, and just overall bad eating habits get us into trouble. We tend to be over-weight, develop serious health issues (diabetes, heart strains, joint pain, depression, anxiety, laziness, etc.), and we simply give up.

This is not a race where you sprint to the finish line. We are in a multi-event long distance marathon, where we take our time. Each meal becomes a winner. So, we may not place first in every event! So, what, we did place.

Life's lessons can be very hard and full of pain. We tend to be stubborn and are only motivated to take a hard look at ourselves when faced with a medical issue. Let's face it, we did not get this way overnight. Yet, we can create a plan to change for the better.

Self-improvement: A critical review of ourselves with a plan to create a new you. This change will happen only when we make that truthful decision to do this for ourselves. Only then will it become a true change, one that we can live with and enjoy our new way of life.

If you try to change for someone else; whether it be family or friends, it seldom sticks. Why, you say? Because it is not in your heart to change. You have not realized the true value or its actual worth for you. Only when you embrace the benefits will you make a conscious decision to change permanently.

Are you important enough to yourself to change for the better?

What value do you see in yourself?

What is your plan? Do you know how to create a plan?

Remember, long-term success is always counted in small steps. The old age saying: "Everyone can eat an elephant," rings true when you start at one bite or one meal.

What motivates you to reach goals? Don't allow small failures to become catastrophic disasters. Everyone stumbles and some even fall. However, the ones who reach the finish line always get back up and take another step. Make the decision to become a healthier eater, be happy in that decision. Stop using "food" as your reward. Instead, add 5 minutes to your walk. Call up a friend. Grabbing a piece of fruit instead of a candy bar is a WIN.

Empower Yourself to Succeed.

After All,

YOU

are the ONE

in

CHARGE!

Date	S M T W T F S	
Breakfast	Amount	Calories (kcal)
	Total	
Snack	Amount	Calories (kcal)
	Total	
Lunch	Amount	Calories (kcal)
	Total	

Snack	Amount	Calories (kcal)
	Total	

Dinner	Amount	Calories (kcal)
	Total	

Snack	Amount	Calories (kcal)
	Total	

Exercise	Duration	Calories burned (kcal)

Water		Fruit & Veges	

Date	S M T W T F S	
Breakfast	Amount	Calories (kcal)
	Total	
Snack	Amount	Calories (kcal)
	Total	
Lunch	Amount	Calories (kcal)
	Total	

Snack	Amount	Calories (kcal)
	Total	
Dinner	Amount	Calories (kcal)
	Total	
Snack	Amount	Calories (kcal)
	Total	
Exercise	Duration	Calories burned (kcal)
Water		Fruit & Veges	

Date	S M T W T F S	
Breakfast	Amount	Calories (kcal)
	Total	
Snack	Amount	Calories (kcal)
	Total	
Lunch	Amount	Calories (kcal)
	Total	

Snack	Amount	Calories (kcal)
	Total	

Dinner	Amount	Calories (kcal)
	Total	

Snack	Amount	Calories (kcal)
	Total	

Exercise	Duration	Calories burned (kcal)

Water		Fruit & Veges	

Date	S M T W T F S	
Breakfast	Amount	Calories (kcal)
	Total	
Snack	Amount	Calories (kcal)
	Total	
Lunch	Amount	Calories (kcal)
	Total	

Snack	Amount	Calories (kcal)
	Total	

Dinner	Amount	Calories (kcal)
	Total	

Snack	Amount	Calories (kcal)
	Total	

Exercise	Duration	Calories burned (kcal)

Water		Fruit & Veges	

Date	S M T W T F S	
Breakfast	Amount	Calories (kcal)
	Total	
Snack	Amount	Calories (kcal)
	Total	
Lunch	Amount	Calories (kcal)
	Total	

Snack	Amount	Calories (kcal)
	Total	

Dinner	Amount	Calories (kcal)
	Total	

Snack	Amount	Calories (kcal)
	Total	

Exercise	Duration	Calories burned (kcal)

Water		Fruit & Veges	

Date		S	M	T	W	T	F	S
Breakfast	Amount	Calories (kcal)						
	Total							
Snack	Amount	Calories (kcal)						
	Total							
Lunch	Amount	Calories (kcal)						
	Total							

Snack	Amount	Calories (kcal)
	Total	

Dinner	Amount	Calories (kcal)
	Total	

Snack	Amount	Calories (kcal)
	Total	

Exercise	Duration	Calories burned (kcal)

Water		Fruit & Veges	

Date		S M T W T F S	
Breakfast		Amount	Calories (kcal)
		Total	
Snack		Amount	Calories (kcal)
		Total	
Lunch		Amount	Calories (kcal)
		Total	

Snack	Amount	Calories (kcal)
	Total	
Dinner	Amount	Calories (kcal)
	Total	
Snack	Amount	Calories (kcal)
	Total	
Exercise	Duration	Calories burned (kcal)
Water		Fruit & Veges	

Date	S M T W T F S	
Breakfast	Amount	Calories (kcal)
	Total	
Snack	Amount	Calories (kcal)
	Total	
Lunch	Amount	Calories (kcal)
	Total	

Snack	Amount	Calories (kcal)
	Total	
Dinner	Amount	Calories (kcal)
	Total	
Snack	Amount	Calories (kcal)
	Total	
Exercise	Duration	Calories burned (kcal)
Water		Fruit & Veges	

Date	S M T W T F S	
Breakfast	Amount	Calories (kcal)
	Total	
Snack	Amount	Calories (kcal)
	Total	
Lunch	Amount	Calories (kcal)
	Total	

Snack	Amount	Calories (kcal)
	Total	

Dinner	Amount	Calories (kcal)
	Total	

Snack	Amount	Calories (kcal)
	Total	

Exercise	Duration	Calories burned (kcal)

Water		Fruit & Veges	

Date	S M T W T F S	
Breakfast	Amount	Calories (kcal)
	Total	
Snack	Amount	Calories (kcal)
	Total	
Lunch	Amount	Calories (kcal)
	Total	

Snack	Amount	Calories (kcal)
	Total	

Dinner	Amount	Calories (kcal)
	Total	

Snack	Amount	Calories (kcal)
	Total	

Exercise	Duration	Calories burned (kcal)

Water									Fruit & Veges								

Date	S M T W T F S	
Breakfast	Amount	Calories (kcal)
	Total	
Snack	Amount	Calories (kcal)
	Total	
Lunch	Amount	Calories (kcal)
	Total	

Snack	Amount	Calories (kcal)
	Total	
Dinner	Amount	Calories (kcal)
	Total	
Snack	Amount	Calories (kcal)
	Total	
Exercise	Duration	Calories burned (kcal)
Water		Fruit & Veges	

Date	S M T W T F S	
Breakfast	Amount	Calories (kcal)
	Total	
Snack	Amount	Calories (kcal)
	Total	
Lunch	Amount	Calories (kcal)
	Total	

Snack	Amount	Calories (kcal)
	Total	

Dinner	Amount	Calories (kcal)
	Total	

Snack	Amount	Calories (kcal)
	Total	

Exercise	Duration	Calories burned (kcal)

Water		Fruit & Veges	

Date		S M T W T F S	
Breakfast		Amount	Calories (kcal)
		Total	
Snack		Amount	Calories (kcal)
		Total	
Lunch		Amount	Calories (kcal)
		Total	

Snack	Amount	Calories (kcal)
	Total	
Dinner	**Amount**	**Calories (kcal)**
	Total	
Snack	**Amount**	**Calories (kcal)**
	Total	
Exercise	**Duration**	**Calories burned (kcal)**

Water								Fruit & Veges							

Date		S M T W T F S	
Breakfast		Amount	Calories (kcal)
		Total	
Snack		Amount	Calories (kcal)
		Total	
Lunch		Amount	Calories (kcal)
		Total	

Snack	Amount	Calories (kcal)
	Total	

Dinner	Amount	Calories (kcal)
	Total	

Snack	Amount	Calories (kcal)
	Total	

Exercise	Duration	Calories burned (kcal)

Water		Fruit & Veges	

Date	S M T W T F S	
Breakfast	Amount	Calories (kcal)
	Total	
Snack	Amount	Calories (kcal)
	Total	
Lunch	Amount	Calories (kcal)
	Total	

Snack	Amount	Calories (kcal)
	Total	

Dinner	Amount	Calories (kcal)
	Total	

Snack	Amount	Calories (kcal)
	Total	

Exercise	Duration	Calories burned (kcal)

Water		Fruit & Veges	

Date	S M T W T F S	
Breakfast	Amount	Calories (kcal)
	Total	
Snack	Amount	Calories (kcal)
	Total	
Lunch	Amount	Calories (kcal)
	Total	

Snack	Amount	Calories (kcal)
	Total	

Dinner	Amount	Calories (kcal)
	Total	

Snack	Amount	Calories (kcal)
	Total	

Exercise	Duration	Calories burned (kcal)

Water		Fruit & Veges	

Date	S M T W T F S	
Breakfast	Amount	Calories (kcal)
	Total	
Snack	Amount	Calories (kcal)
	Total	
Lunch	Amount	Calories (kcal)
	Total	

Snack	Amount	Calories (kcal)
	Total	

Dinner	Amount	Calories (kcal)
	Total	

Snack	Amount	Calories (kcal)
	Total	

Exercise	Duration	Calories burned (kcal)

Water		Fruit & Veges	

Date	S M T W T F S	
Breakfast	Amount	Calories (kcal)
	Total	
Snack	Amount	Calories (kcal)
	Total	
Lunch	Amount	Calories (kcal)
	Total	

Snack	Amount	Calories (kcal)
	Total	

Dinner	Amount	Calories (kcal)
	Total	

Snack	Amount	Calories (kcal)
	Total	

Exercise	Duration	Calories burned (kcal)

Water		Fruit & Veges	

Date	S M T W T F S	
Breakfast	Amount	Calories (kcal)
	Total	
Snack	Amount	Calories (kcal)
	Total	
Lunch	Amount	Calories (kcal)
	Total	

Snack	Amount	Calories (kcal)
	Total	
Dinner	Amount	Calories (kcal)
	Total	
Snack	Amount	Calories (kcal)
	Total	
Exercise	Duration	Calories burned (kcal)
Water									Fruit & Veges								

Date	S	M	T	W	T	F	S	
Breakfast	Amount							Calories (kcal)
	Total							
Snack	Amount							Calories (kcal)
	Total							
Lunch	Amount							Calories (kcal)
	Total							

Snack	Amount	Calories (kcal)
	Total	

Dinner	Amount	Calories (kcal)
	Total	

Snack	Amount	Calories (kcal)
	Total	

Exercise	Duration	Calories burned (kcal)

Water		Fruit & Veges	

Date	S M T W T F S	
Breakfast	Amount	Calories (kcal)
	Total	
Snack	Amount	Calories (kcal)
	Total	
Lunch	Amount	Calories (kcal)
	Total	

Snack	Amount	Calories (kcal)
	Total	
Dinner	Amount	Calories (kcal)
	Total	
Snack	Amount	Calories (kcal)
	Total	
Exercise	Duration	Calories burned (kcal)
Water									Fruit & Veges								

Date	S M T W T F S	
Breakfast	Amount	Calories (kcal)
	Total	
Snack	Amount	Calories (kcal)
	Total	
Lunch	Amount	Calories (kcal)
	Total	

Snack	Amount	Calories (kcal)
	Total	

Dinner	Amount	Calories (kcal)
	Total	

Snack	Amount	Calories (kcal)
	Total	

Exercise	Duration	Calories burned (kcal)

Water									Fruit & Veges								

Date	S M T W T F S	
Breakfast	Amount	Calories (kcal)
	Total	
Snack	Amount	Calories (kcal)
	Total	
Lunch	Amount	Calories (kcal)
	Total	

Snack	Amount	Calories (kcal)
	Total	
Dinner	**Amount**	**Calories (kcal)**
	Total	
Snack	**Amount**	**Calories (kcal)**
	Total	
Exercise	**Duration**	**Calories burned (kcal)**
Water		Fruit & Veges	

Date	S M T W T F S	
Breakfast	Amount	Calories (kcal)
	Total	
Snack	Amount	Calories (kcal)
	Total	
Lunch	Amount	Calories (kcal)
	Total	

Snack	Amount	Calories (kcal)
	Total	

Dinner	Amount	Calories (kcal)
	Total	

Snack	Amount	Calories (kcal)
	Total	

Exercise	Duration	Calories burned (kcal)

Water		Fruit & Veges	

Date	S M T W T F S	
Breakfast	Amount	Calories (kcal)
	Total	
Snack	Amount	Calories (kcal)
	Total	
Lunch	Amount	Calories (kcal)
	Total	

Snack	Amount	Calories (kcal)
	Total	

Dinner	Amount	Calories (kcal)
	Total	

Snack	Amount	Calories (kcal)
	Total	

Exercise	Duration	Calories burned (kcal)

Water		Fruit & Veges	

Date	S M T W T F S	
Breakfast	**Amount**	**Calories (kcal)**
	Total	
Snack	**Amount**	**Calories (kcal)**
	Total	
Lunch	**Amount**	**Calories (kcal)**
	Total	

Snack	Amount	Calories (kcal)
	Total	
Dinner	Amount	Calories (kcal)
	Total	
Snack	Amount	Calories (kcal)
	Total	
Exercise	Duration	Calories burned (kcal)
Water		Fruit & Veges	

Date	S M T W T F S	
Breakfast	**Amount**	**Calories (kcal)**
	Total	
Snack	**Amount**	**Calories (kcal)**
	Total	
Lunch	**Amount**	**Calories (kcal)**
	Total	

Snack	Amount	Calories (kcal)
	Total	

Dinner	Amount	Calories (kcal)
	Total	

Snack	Amount	Calories (kcal)
	Total	

Exercise	Duration	Calories burned (kcal)

Water		Fruit & Veges	

Date	S M T W T F S	
Breakfast	Amount	Calories (kcal)
	Total	
Snack	Amount	Calories (kcal)
	Total	
Lunch	Amount	Calories (kcal)
	Total	

Snack	Amount	Calories (kcal)
	Total	

Dinner	Amount	Calories (kcal)
	Total	

Snack	Amount	Calories (kcal)
	Total	

Exercise	Duration	Calories burned (kcal)

Water		Fruit & Veges	

Date	S M T W T F S	
Breakfast	Amount	Calories (kcal)
	Total	
Snack	Amount	Calories (kcal)
	Total	
Lunch	Amount	Calories (kcal)
	Total	

Snack	Amount	Calories (kcal)
	Total	
Dinner	Amount	Calories (kcal)
	Total	
Snack	Amount	Calories (kcal)
	Total	
Exercise	Duration	Calories burned (kcal)
Water		Fruit & Veges	

Date	S M T W T F S	
Breakfast	Amount	Calories (kcal)
	Total	
Snack	Amount	Calories (kcal)
	Total	
Lunch	Amount	Calories (kcal)
	Total	

Snack	Amount	Calories (kcal)
	Total	

Dinner	Amount	Calories (kcal)
	Total	

Snack	Amount	Calories (kcal)
	Total	

Exercise	Duration	Calories burned (kcal)

Water		Fruit & Veges	

Date	S M T W T F S	
Breakfast	Amount	Calories (kcal)
	Total	
Snack	Amount	Calories (kcal)
	Total	
Lunch	Amount	Calories (kcal)
	Total	

Snack	Amount	Calories (kcal)
	Total	
Dinner	Amount	Calories (kcal)
	Total	
Snack	Amount	Calories (kcal)
	Total	
Exercise	Duration	Calories burned (kcal)
Water		Fruit & Veges	

The first month is completed!

How did you do?

Did you achieve your goal?

How has your plans changed through your journey?

If you included or added exercise, what change did it make?

Did your foods change or how you prepared your food ?

What goals have you set for the next 30 days?

My Changing Body

	Second Month Challenge			
Measurements	Week 1	Week 2	Week 3	Week 4
Neck				
Right Upper				
Left Upper Arm				
Right Wrist				
Left Wrist				
Chest				
Bust				
Midriff				
Natural Waist				
Abdomen				
Hips				
Buttocks				
Upper Thigh				
Middle Thigh				
Lower Thigh				
Above Knee				
Calf				
Ankle				
Starting				
Goal Weight				

Did you power through your ups and downs? What did you do?

DO NOT get discouraged.

Change up your food selections, add a different type of exercise, and most of all –

Are you Drinking YOUR WATER!

Date	S M T W T F S	
Breakfast	Amount	Calories (kcal)
	Total	
Snack	Amount	Calories (kcal)
	Total	
Lunch	Amount	Calories (kcal)
	Total	

Snack	Amount	Calories (kcal)
	Total	
Dinner	Amount	Calories (kcal)
	Total	
Snack	Amount	Calories (kcal)
	Total	
Exercise	Duration	Calories burned (kcal)

Water							Fruit & Veges							

Date	S M T W T F S	
Breakfast	Amount	Calories (kcal)
	Total	
Snack	Amount	Calories (kcal)
	Total	
Lunch	Amount	Calories (kcal)
	Total	

Snack	Amount	Calories (kcal)
	Total	
Dinner	Amount	Calories (kcal)
	Total	
Snack	Amount	Calories (kcal)
	Total	
Exercise	Duration	Calories burned (kcal)
Water		Fruit & Veges	

Date	S M T W T F S	
Breakfast	Amount	Calories (kcal)
	Total	
Snack	Amount	Calories (kcal)
	Total	
Lunch	Amount	Calories (kcal)
	Total	

Snack	Amount	Calories (kcal)
	Total	

Dinner	Amount	Calories (kcal)
	Total	

Snack	Amount	Calories (kcal)
	Total	

Exercise	Duration	Calories burned (kcal)

Water		Fruit & Veges	

Date	S M T W T F S	
Breakfast	Amount	Calories (kcal)
	Total	
Snack	Amount	Calories (kcal)
	Total	
Lunch	Amount	Calories (kcal)
	Total	

Snack	Amount	Calories (kcal)
	Total	
Dinner	**Amount**	**Calories (kcal)**
	Total	
Snack	**Amount**	**Calories (kcal)**
	Total	
Exercise	**Duration**	**Calories burned (kcal)**
Water								Fruit & Veges								

Date	S M T W T F S	
Breakfast	Amount	Calories (kcal)
	Total	
Snack	Amount	Calories (kcal)
	Total	
Lunch	Amount	Calories (kcal)
	S M T W T F S	
	Total	

Snack	Amount	Calories (kcal)
	Total	
Dinner	Amount	Calories (kcal)
	Total	
Snack	Amount	Calories (kcal)
	Total	
Exercise	Duration	Calories burned (kcal)
Water		Fruit & Veges	

Date	S M T W T F S	
Breakfast	Amount	Calories (kcal)
	Total	
Snack	Amount	Calories (kcal)
	Total	
Lunch	Amount	Calories (kcal)
	Total	

Snack	Amount	Calories (kcal)
	Total	

Dinner	Amount	Calories (kcal)
	Total	

Snack	Amount	Calories (kcal)
	Total	

Exercise	Duration	Calories burned (kcal)

Water		Fruit & Veges	

Date	S M T W T F S	
Breakfast	Amount	Calories (kcal)
	Total	
Snack	Amount	Calories (kcal)
	Total	
Lunch	Amount	Calories (kcal)
	Total	

Snack	Amount	Calories (kcal)
	Total	
Dinner	Amount	Calories (kcal)
	Total	
Snack	Amount	Calories (kcal)
	Total	
Exercise	Duration	Calories burned (kcal)
Water									Fruit & Veges									

Date	S M T W T F S	
Breakfast	Amount	Calories (kcal)
	Total	
Snack	Amount	Calories (kcal)
	Total	
Lunch	Amount	Calories (kcal)
	Total	

Snack	Amount	Calories (kcal)
	Total	

Dinner	Amount	Calories (kcal)
	Total	

Snack	Amount	Calories (kcal)
	Total	

Exercise	Duration	Calories burned (kcal)

Water		Fruit & Veges	

Date	S M T W T F S	
Breakfast	Amount	Calories (kcal)
	Total	
Snack	Amount	Calories (kcal)
	Total	
Lunch	Amount	Calories (kcal)
	Total	

Snack	Amount	Calories (kcal)
	Total	

Dinner	Amount	Calories (kcal)
	Total	

Snack	Amount	Calories (kcal)
	Total	

Exercise	Duration	Calories burned (kcal)

Water		Fruit & Veges	

Date	S M T W T F S	
Breakfast	Amount	Calories (kcal)
	Total	
Snack	Amount	Calories (kcal)
	Total	
Lunch	Amount	Calories (kcal)
	Total	

Snack	Amount	Calories (kcal)
	Total	

Dinner	Amount	Calories (kcal)
	Total	

Snack	Amount	Calories (kcal)
	Total	

Exercise	Duration	Calories burned (kcal)

Water		Fruit & Veges	

Date	S M T W T F S	
Breakfast	Amount	Calories (kcal)
	Total	
Snack	Amount	Calories (kcal)
	Total	
Lunch	Amount	Calories (kcal)
	Total	

Snack	Amount	Calories (kcal)
	Total	

Dinner	Amount	Calories (kcal)
	Total	

Snack	Amount	Calories (kcal)
	Total	

Exercise	Duration	Calories burned (kcal)

Water		Fruit & Veges	

Date	S M T W T F S	
Breakfast	Amount	Calories (kcal)
	Total	
Snack	Amount	Calories (kcal)
	Total	
Lunch	Amount	Calories (kcal)
	Total	

Snack	Amount	Calories (kcal)
	Total	

Dinner	Amount	Calories (kcal)
	Total	

Snack	Amount	Calories (kcal)
	Total	

Exercise	Duration	Calories burned (kcal)

Water		Fruit & Veges	

Date	S M T W T F S	
Breakfast	Amount	Calories (kcal)
	Total	
Snack	Amount	Calories (kcal)
	Total	
Lunch	Amount	Calories (kcal)
	Total	

Snack	Amount	Calories (kcal)
	Total	
Dinner	Amount	Calories (kcal)
	Total	
Snack	Amount	Calories (kcal)
	Total	
Exercise	Duration	Calories burned (kcal)
Water								Fruit & Veges								

Date	S M T W T F S	
Breakfast	Amount	Calories (kcal)
	Total	
Snack	Amount	Calories (kcal)
	Total	
Lunch	Amount	Calories (kcal)
	Total	

Snack	Amount	Calories (kcal)
	Total	

Dinner	Amount	Calories (kcal)
	Total	

Snack	Amount	Calories (kcal)
	Total	

Exercise	Duration	Calories burned (kcal)

Water		Fruit & Veges	

Date	S M T W T F S	
Breakfast	Amount	Calories (kcal)
	Total	
Snack	Amount	Calories (kcal)
	Total	
Lunch	Amount	Calories (kcal)
	Total	

Snack	Amount	Calories (kcal)
	Total	

Dinner	Amount	Calories (kcal)
	Total	

Snack	Amount	Calories (kcal)
	Total	

Exercise	Duration	Calories burned (kcal)

Water		Fruit & Veges	

Date	S M T W T F S	
Breakfast	Amount	Calories (kcal)
	Total	
Snack	Amount	Calories (kcal)
	Total	
Lunch	Amount	Calories (kcal)
	Total	

Snack	Amount	Calories (kcal)
	Total	
Dinner	Amount	Calories (kcal)
	Total	
Snack	Amount	Calories (kcal)
	Total	
Exercise	Duration	Calories burned (kcal)
Water		Fruit & Veges	

Date	S M T W T F S	
Breakfast	Amount	Calories (kcal)
	Total	
Snack	Amount	Calories (kcal)
	Total	
Lunch	Amount	Calories (kcal)
	Total	

Snack	Amount	Calories (kcal)
	Total	

Dinner	Amount	Calories (kcal)
	Total	

Snack	Amount	Calories (kcal)
	Total	

Exercise	Duration	Calories burned (kcal)

Water									Fruit & Veges							

Date	S M T W T F S	
Breakfast	Amount	Calories (kcal)
	Total	
Snack	Amount	Calories (kcal)
	Total	
Lunch	Amount	Calories (kcal)
	Total	

Snack	Amount	Calories (kcal)
	Total	
Dinner	Amount	Calories (kcal)
	Total	
Snack	Amount	Calories (kcal)
	Total	
Exercise	Duration	Calories burned (kcal)
Water		Fruit & Veges	

Date	S M T W T F S	
Breakfast	Amount	Calories (kcal)
	Total	
Snack	Amount	Calories (kcal)
	Total	
Lunch	Amount	Calories (kcal)
	Total	

Snack	Amount	Calories (kcal)
	Total	

Dinner	Amount	Calories (kcal)
	Total	

Snack	Amount	Calories (kcal)
	Total	

Exercise	Duration	Calories burned (kcal)

Water		Fruit & Veges	

Date			S	M	T	W	T	F	S
Breakfast			Amount				Calories (kcal)		
			Total						
Snack			Amount				Calories (kcal)		
			Total						
Lunch			Amount				Calories (kcal)		
			S	M	T	W	T	F	S
			Total						

Snack	Amount	Calories (kcal)
	Total	

Dinner	Amount	Calories (kcal)
	Total	

Snack	Amount	Calories (kcal)
	Total	

Exercise	Duration	Calories burned (kcal)

Water		Fruit & Veges	

Date	S	M	T	W	T	F	S

Breakfast	Amount	Calories (kcal)
	Total	

Snack	Amount	Calories (kcal)
	Total	

Lunch	Amount	Calories (kcal)
	Total	

Snack	Amount	Calories (kcal)
	Total	
Dinner	Amount	Calories (kcal)
	Total	
Snack	Amount	Calories (kcal)
	Total	
Exercise	Duration	Calories burned (kcal)
Water		Fruit & Veges	

Date	S M T W T F S	
Breakfast	Amount	Calories (kcal)
	Total	
Snack	Amount	Calories (kcal)
	Total	
Lunch	Amount	Calories (kcal)
	Total	

Snack	Amount	Calories (kcal)
	Total	

Dinner	Amount	Calories (kcal)
	Total	

Snack	Amount	Calories (kcal)
	Total	

Exercise	Duration	Calories burned (kcal)

Water		Fruit & Veges	

Date	S M T W T F S	
Breakfast	Amount	Calories (kcal)
	Total	
Snack	Amount	Calories (kcal)
	Total	
Lunch	Amount	Calories (kcal)
	Total	

Snack	Amount	Calories (kcal)
	Total	

Dinner	Amount	Calories (kcal)
	Total	

Snack	Amount	Calories (kcal)
	Total	

Exercise	Duration	Calories burned (kcal)

Water		Fruit & Veges	

Date		S	M	T	W	T	F	S
Breakfast		Amount			Calories (kcal)			
		Total						
Snack		Amount			Calories (kcal)			
		Total						
Lunch		Amount			Calories (kcal)			
		Total						

Snack	Amount	Calories (kcal)
	Total	

Dinner	Amount	Calories (kcal)
	Total	

Snack	Amount	Calories (kcal)
	Total	

Exercise	Duration	Calories burned (kcal)

Water		Fruit & Veges	

Date	S M T W T F S	
Breakfast	Amount	Calories (kcal)
	Total	
Snack	Amount	Calories (kcal)
	Total	
Lunch	Amount	Calories (kcal)
	Total	

Snack	Amount	Calories (kcal)
	Total	

Dinner	Amount	Calories (kcal)
	Total	

Snack	Amount	Calories (kcal)
	Total	

Exercise	Duration	Calories burned (kcal)

Water		Fruit & Veges	

Date	S M T W T F S	
Breakfast	Amount	Calories (kcal)
	Total	
Snack	Amount	Calories (kcal)
	Total	
Lunch	Amount	Calories (kcal)
	Total	

Snack	Amount	Calories (kcal)
	Total	

Dinner	Amount	Calories (kcal)
	Total	

Snack	Amount	Calories (kcal)
	Total	

Exercise	Duration	Calories burned (kcal)

Water		Fruit & Veges	

Date	S M T W T F S	
Breakfast	**Amount**	**Calories (kcal)**
	Total	
Snack	**Amount**	**Calories (kcal)**
	Total	
Lunch	**Amount**	**Calories (kcal)**
	Total	

Snack	Amount	Calories (kcal)
	Total	

Dinner	Amount	Calories (kcal)
	Total	

Snack	Amount	Calories (kcal)
	Total	

Exercise	Duration	Calories burned (kcal)

Water		Fruit & Veges	

Date		S	M	T	W	T	F	S
Breakfast	Amount	Calories (kcal)						
	Total							
Snack	Amount	Calories (kcal)						
	Total							
Lunch	Amount	Calories (kcal)						
	Total							

Snack	Amount	Calories (kcal)
	Total	
Dinner	Amount	Calories (kcal)
	Total	
Snack	Amount	Calories (kcal)
	Total	
Exercise	Duration	Calories burned (kcal)
Water								Fruit & Veges								

Date	S M T W T F S	
Breakfast	Amount	Calories (kcal)
	Total	
Snack	Amount	Calories (kcal)
	Total	
Lunch	Amount	Calories (kcal)
	Total	

Snack	Amount	Calories (kcal)
	Total	

Dinner	Amount	Calories (kcal)
	Total	

Snack	Amount	Calories (kcal)
	Total	

Exercise	Duration	Calories burned (kcal)

Water		Fruit & Veges	

Date	S M T W T F S	
Breakfast	Amount	Calories (kcal)
	Total	
Snack	Amount	Calories (kcal)
	Total	
Lunch	Amount	Calories (kcal)
	Total	

Snack	Amount	Calories (kcal)
	Total	
Dinner	Amount	Calories (kcal)
	Total	
Snack	Amount	Calories (kcal)
	Total	
Exercise	Duration	Calories burned (kcal)
Water		Fruit & Veges	

Date	S M T W T F S	
Breakfast	Amount	Calories (kcal)
	Total	
Snack	Amount	Calories (kcal)
	Total	
Lunch	Amount	Calories (kcal)
	Total	

Snack	Amount	Calories (kcal)
	Total	

Dinner	Amount	Calories (kcal)
	Total	

Snack	Amount	Calories (kcal)
	Total	

Exercise	Duration	Calories burned (kcal)

Water		Fruit & Veges	

The second month is completed!

How did you do?

Did you achieve your goal?

How has your plans changed through your journey?

If you included or added exercise, what change did it make?

Did your foods change or how you prepared your food ?

What goal have you set for the next 30 days?

My Changing Body

Third Month Challenge				
Measurements	Week 1	Week 2	Week 3	Week 4
Neck				
Right Upper				
Left Upper Arm				
Right Wrist				
Left Wrist				
Chest				
Bust				
Midriff				
Natural Waist				
Abdomen				
Hips				
Buttocks				
Upper Thigh				
Middle Thigh				
Lower Thigh				
Above Knee				
Calf				
Ankle				
Starting				
Goal Weight				

Did you power through your ups and downs? What did you do?

DO NOT get discouraged.

Change up your food selections, add a different type of exercise, and most of all –

Are you Drinking YOUR WATER!

Date		S　M　T　W　T　F　S	
Breakfast		Amount	Calories (kcal)
		Total	
Snack		Amount	Calories (kcal)
		Total	
Lunch		Amount	Calories (kcal)
		Total	

Snack	Amount	Calories (kcal)
	Total	

Dinner	Amount	Calories (kcal)
	Total	

Snack	Amount	Calories (kcal)
	Total	

Exercise	Duration	Calories burned (kcal)

Water		Fruit & Veges	

Date	S M T W T F S	
Breakfast	Amount	Calories (kcal)
	Total	
Snack	Amount	Calories (kcal)
	Total	
Lunch	Amount	Calories (kcal)
	Total	

Snack	Amount	Calories (kcal)
	Total	

Dinner	Amount	Calories (kcal)
	Total	

Snack	Amount	Calories (kcal)
	Total	

Exercise	Duration	Calories burned (kcal)

Water		Fruit & Veges	

Date	S	M	T	W	T	F	S
Breakfast	Amount			Calories (kcal)			
	Total						
Snack	Amount			Calories (kcal)			
	Total						
Lunch	Amount			Calories (kcal)			
	Total						

Snack	Amount	Calories (kcal)
	Total	
Dinner	Amount	Calories (kcal)
	Total	
Snack	Amount	Calories (kcal)
	Total	
Exercise	Duration	Calories burned (kcal)
Water		Fruit & Veges	

Date		S	M	T	W	T	F	S
Breakfast		Amount		Calories (kcal)				
		Total						
Snack		Amount		Calories (kcal)				
		Total						
Lunch		Amount		Calories (kcal)				
		Total						

Snack	Amount	Calories (kcal)
	Total	

Dinner	Amount	Calories (kcal)
	Total	

Snack	Amount	Calories (kcal)
	Total	

Exercise	Duration	Calories burned (kcal)

Water		Fruit & Veges	

Date		S M T W T F S	
Breakfast		Amount	Calories (kcal)
		Total	
Snack		Amount	Calories (kcal)
		Total	
Lunch		Amount	Calories (kcal)
		Total	

Snack	Amount	Calories (kcal)
	Total	
Dinner	Amount	Calories (kcal)
	Total	
Snack	Amount	Calories (kcal)
	Total	
Exercise	Duration	Calories burned (kcal)
Water		Fruit & Veges

Date	S M T W T F S	
Breakfast	Amount	Calories (kcal)
	Total	
Snack	Amount	Calories (kcal)
	Total	
Lunch	Amount	Calories (kcal)
	Total	

Snack	Amount	Calories (kcal)
	Total	

Dinner	Amount	Calories (kcal)
	Total	

Snack	Amount	Calories (kcal)
	Total	

Exercise	Duration	Calories burned (kcal)

Water		Fruit & Veges	

Date	S M T W T F S	
Breakfast	Amount	Calories (kcal)
	Total	
Snack	Amount	Calories (kcal)
	Total	
Lunch	Amount	Calories (kcal)
	Total	

Snack	Amount	Calories (kcal)
	Total	

Dinner	Amount	Calories (kcal)
	Total	

Snack	Amount	Calories (kcal)
	Total	

Exercise	Duration	Calories burned (kcal)

Water		Fruit & Veges	

Date	S M T W T F S	
Breakfast	Amount	Calories (kcal)
	Total	
Snack	Amount	Calories (kcal)
	Total	
Lunch	Amount	Calories (kcal)
	Total	

Snack	Amount	Calories (kcal)
	Total	

Dinner	Amount	Calories (kcal)
	Total	

Snack	Amount	Calories (kcal)
	Total	

Exercise	Duration	Calories burned (kcal)

Water		Fruit & Veges	

Date	S M T W T F S	
Breakfast	Amount	Calories (kcal)
	Total	
Snack	Amount	Calories (kcal)
	Total	
Lunch	Amount	Calories (kcal)
	Total	

Snack	Amount	Calories (kcal)
	Total	
Dinner	Amount	Calories (kcal)
	Total	
Snack	Amount	Calories (kcal)
	Total	
Exercise	Duration	Calories burned (kcal)
Water		Fruit & Veges	

Date	S M T W T F S	
Breakfast	Amount	Calories (kcal)
	Total	
Snack	Amount	Calories (kcal)
	Total	
Lunch	Amount	Calories (kcal)
	Total	

Snack	Amount	Calories (kcal)
	Total	

Dinner	Amount	Calories (kcal)
	Total	

Snack	Amount	Calories (kcal)
	Total	

Exercise	Duration	Calories burned (kcal)

Water		Fruit & Veges	

Date	S	M	T	W	T	F	S	
Breakfast	Amount							Calories (kcal)
	Total							
Snack	Amount							Calories (kcal)
	Total							
Lunch	Amount							Calories (kcal)
	Total							

Snack	Amount	Calories (kcal)
	Total	
Dinner	Amount	Calories (kcal)
	Total	
Snack	Amount	Calories (kcal)
	Total	
Exercise	Duration	Calories burned (kcal)
Water								Fruit & Veges								

Date	S M T W T F S	
Breakfast	Amount	Calories (kcal)
	Total	
Snack	Amount	Calories (kcal)
	Total	
Lunch	Amount	Calories (kcal)
	Total	

Snack	Amount	Calories (kcal)
	Total	

Dinner	Amount	Calories (kcal)
	Total	

Snack	Amount	Calories (kcal)
	Total	

Exercise	Duration	Calories burned (kcal)

Water		Fruit & Veges	

Date	S M T W T F S	
Breakfast	Amount	Calories (kcal)
	Total	
Snack	Amount	Calories (kcal)
	Total	
Lunch	Amount	Calories (kcal)
	Total	

Snack	Amount	Calories (kcal)
	Total	
Dinner	Amount	Calories (kcal)
	Total	
Snack	Amount	Calories (kcal)
	Total	
Exercise	Duration	Calories burned (kcal)
Water		Fruit & Veges	

Date	S M T W T F S	
Breakfast	Amount	Calories (kcal)
	Total	
Snack	Amount	Calories (kcal)
	Total	
Lunch	Amount	Calories (kcal)
	Total	

Snack	Amount	Calories (kcal)
	Total	

Dinner	Amount	Calories (kcal)
	Total	

Snack	Amount	Calories (kcal)
	Total	

Exercise	Duration	Calories burned (kcal)

Water		Fruit & Veges	

Date		S M T W T F S	
Breakfast		Amount	Calories (kcal)
		Total	
Snack		Amount	Calories (kcal)
		Total	
Lunch		Amount	Calories (kcal)
		Total	

Snack	Amount	Calories (kcal)
	Total	

Dinner	Amount	Calories (kcal)
	Total	

Snack	Amount	Calories (kcal)
	Total	

Exercise	Duration	Calories burned (kcal)

Water		Fruit & Veges	

Date		S M T W T F S	
Breakfast		Amount	Calories (kcal)
		Total	
Snack		Amount	Calories (kcal)
		Total	
Lunch		Amount	Calories (kcal)
		Total	

Snack	Amount	Calories (kcal)
	Total	

Dinner	Amount	Calories (kcal)
	Total	

Snack	Amount	Calories (kcal)
	Total	

Exercise	Duration	Calories burned (kcal)

Water		Fruit & Veges	

Date	S M T W T F S	
Breakfast	Amount	Calories (kcal)
	Total	
Snack	Amount	Calories (kcal)
	Total	
Lunch	Amount	Calories (kcal)
	Total	

Snack	Amount	Calories (kcal)
	Total	

Dinner	Amount	Calories (kcal)
	Total	

Snack	Amount	Calories (kcal)
	Total	

Exercise	Duration	Calories burned (kcal)

Water		Fruit & Veges	

Date	S M T W T F S	
Breakfast	Amount	Calories (kcal)
	Total	
Snack	Amount	Calories (kcal)
	Total	
Lunch	Amount	Calories (kcal)
	Total	

Snack	Amount	Calories (kcal)
	Total	
Dinner	Amount	Calories (kcal)
	Total	
Snack	Amount	Calories (kcal)
	Total	
Exercise	Duration	Calories burned (kcal)
Water		Fruit & Veges	

Date		S M T W T F S	
Breakfast		Amount	Calories (kcal)
		Total	
Snack		Amount	Calories (kcal)
		Total	
Lunch		Amount	Calories (kcal)
		Total	

Snack	Amount	Calories (kcal)
	Total	

Dinner	Amount	Calories (kcal)
	Total	

Snack	Amount	Calories (kcal)
	Total	

Exercise	Duration	Calories burned (kcal)

Water		Fruit & Veges	

Date	S M T W T F S	
Breakfast	Amount	Calories (kcal)
	Total	
Snack	Amount	Calories (kcal)
	Total	
Lunch	Amount	Calories (kcal)
	Total	

Snack	Amount	Calories (kcal)
	Total	

Dinner	Amount	Calories (kcal)
	Total	

Snack	Amount	Calories (kcal)
	Total	

Exercise	Duration	Calories burned (kcal)

Water		Fruit & Veges	

Date	S M T W T F S	
Breakfast	Amount	Calories (kcal)
	Total	
Snack	Amount	Calories (kcal)
	Total	
Lunch	Amount	Calories (kcal)
	Total	

Snack	Amount	Calories (kcal)
	Total	
Dinner	Amount	Calories (kcal)
	Total	
Snack	Amount	Calories (kcal)
	Total	
Exercise	Duration	Calories burned (kcal)
Water		Fruit & Veges	

Date	S M T W T F S	
Breakfast	Amount	Calories (kcal)
	Total	
Snack	Amount	Calories (kcal)
	Total	
Lunch	Amount	Calories (kcal)
	Total	

Snack	Amount	Calories (kcal)
	Total	

Dinner	Amount	Calories (kcal)
	Total	

Snack	Amount	Calories (kcal)
	Total	

Exercise	Duration	Calories burned (kcal)

Water		Fruit & Veges	

Date	S M T W T F S	
Breakfast	Amount	Calories (kcal)
	Total	
Snack	Amount	Calories (kcal)
	Total	
Lunch	Amount	Calories (kcal)
	Total	

Snack	Amount	Calories (kcal)
	Total	

Dinner	Amount	Calories (kcal)
	Total	

Snack	Amount	Calories (kcal)
	Total	

Exercise	Duration	Calories burned (kcal)

Water		Fruit & Veges	

Date	S	M	T	W	T	F	S
Breakfast	Amount		Calories (kcal)				
	Total						
Snack	Amount		Calories (kcal)				
	Total						
Lunch	Amount		Calories (kcal)				
	Total						

Snack	Amount	Calories (kcal)
	Total	
Dinner	Amount	Calories (kcal)
	Total	
Snack	Amount	Calories (kcal)
	Total	
Exercise	Duration	Calories burned (kcal)
Water		Fruit & Veges	

Date	S M T W T F S	
Breakfast	Amount	Calories (kcal)
	Total	
Snack	Amount	Calories (kcal)
	Total	
Lunch	Amount	Calories (kcal)
	Total	

Snack	Amount	Calories (kcal)
	Total	
Dinner	Amount	Calories (kcal)
	Total	
Snack	Amount	Calories (kcal)
	Total	
Exercise	Duration	Calories burned (kcal)
Water		Fruit & Veges	

Date	S M T W T F S	
Breakfast	Amount	Calories (kcal)
	Total	
Snack	Amount	Calories (kcal)
	Total	
Lunch	Amount	Calories (kcal)
	Total	

Snack	Amount	Calories (kcal)
	Total	

Dinner	Amount	Calories (kcal)
	Total	

Snack	Amount	Calories (kcal)
	Total	

Exercise	Duration	Calories burned (kcal)

Water		Fruit & Veges	

Date	S M T W T F S	
Breakfast	Amount	Calories (kcal)
	Total	
Snack	Amount	Calories (kcal)
	Total	
Lunch	Amount	Calories (kcal)
	Total	

Snack	Amount	Calories (kcal)
	Total	

Dinner	Amount	Calories (kcal)
	Total	

Snack	Amount	Calories (kcal)
	Total	

Exercise	Duration	Calories burned (kcal)

Water		Fruit & Veges	

Date		S　M　T　W　T　F　S	
Breakfast		Amount	Calories (kcal)
		Total	
Snack		Amount	Calories (kcal)
		Total	
Lunch		Amount	Calories (kcal)
		Total	

Snack	Amount	Calories (kcal)
	Total	

Dinner	Amount	Calories (kcal)
	Total	

Snack	Amount	Calories (kcal)
	Total	

Exercise	Duration	Calories burned (kcal)

Water		Fruit & Veges	

Date	S M T W T F S	
Breakfast	Amount	Calories (kcal)
	Total	
Snack	Amount	Calories (kcal)
	Total	
Lunch	Amount	Calories (kcal)
	Total	

Snack	Amount	Calories (kcal)
	Total	

Dinner	Amount	Calories (kcal)
	Total	

Snack	Amount	Calories (kcal)
	Total	

Exercise	Duration	Calories burned (kcal)

Water									Fruit & Veges								

Date	S M T W T F S	
Breakfast	Amount	Calories (kcal)
	Total	
Snack	Amount	Calories (kcal)
	Total	
Lunch	Amount	Calories (kcal)
	Total	

Snack	Amount	Calories (kcal)
	Total	
Dinner	Amount	Calories (kcal)
	Total	
Snack	Amount	Calories (kcal)
	Total	
Exercise	Duration	Calories burned (kcal)
Water		Fruit & Veges	

Date		S M T W T F S	
Breakfast		Amount	Calories (kcal)
		Total	
Snack		Amount	Calories (kcal)
		Total	
Lunch		Amount	Calories (kcal)
		Total	

Snack	Amount	Calories (kcal)
	Total	

Dinner	Amount	Calories (kcal)
	Total	

Snack	Amount	Calories (kcal)
	Total	

Exercise	Duration	Calories burned (kcal)

Water		Fruit & Veges	

Date	S M T W T F S	
Breakfast	Amount	Calories (kcal)
	Total	
Snack	Amount	Calories (kcal)
	Total	
Lunch	Amount	Calories (kcal)
	Total	

Snack	Amount	Calories (kcal)
	Total	

Dinner	Amount	Calories (kcal)
	Total	

Snack	Amount	Calories (kcal)
	Total	

Exercise	Duration	Calories burned (kcal)

Water		Fruit & Veges	

The third month is completed!

How did you do?

Did you achieve your goal?

How has your plans changed through your journey?

If you included or added exercise, what change did it make?

Did your foods change or how you prepared your food?

What goal have you set for the next 30 days?

Notes

Thank you for staying with this challenge. I hope you achieved success. And, most of all, you learned how your body processes the food you eat and how to manage your weight to stay healthy.

I needed something that was inspiring, informative, and created accountability for me to stay focused on my weight loss journey. So, I created this journal.

I hope you continue to be inspired and stay focused along your weight loss journey.

Sincerely,

Janet Bullard

www.janetbullard.com

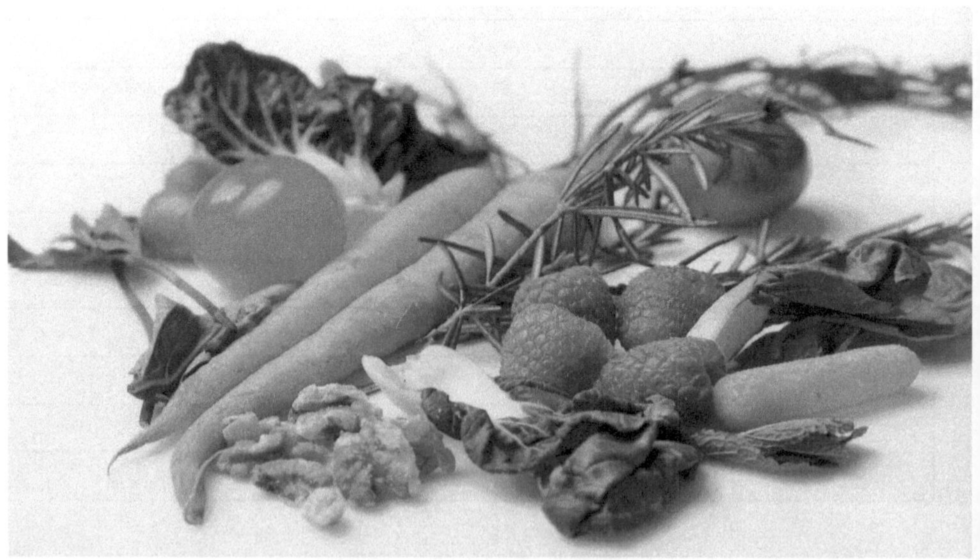